Easy Yoga For Pregnancy: Pelvic Floor Poses To Boost Fertility For Expecting Mums.

By

Rose S. Rogers

INTRODUCTION

Pregnancy is an amazing experience full of excitement, joy, and profound changes. It's a time when your body, mind, and spirit unite in anticipation of the wonderful advent of your child. Yoga may be a trusted partner along this path, providing not just physical advantages but also a profound sense of well-being.

In this guide, we'll look at "Easy Yoga for Pregnancy: Pelvic Floor Poses to Boost Fertility for Expecting Moms." This book is intended to accompany you on this great journey, whether you are a first-time mom-to-be or have already experienced the pleasures of motherhood.

We'll look at the many benefits of yoga during pregnancy, from improving physical flexibility and strength to promoting emotional balance and relaxation. We'll concentrate on pelvic floor postures in particular, which are important for overall health and fertility.

We hope to provide you with a tool set to handle the challenges and joys of pregnancy by combining yoga's gentle yet powerful postures with mindfulness practices. Whether you want to improve your fertility, strengthen your pelvic floor, or simply find peace in the midst of the changes, our journey through simple yoga for pregnancy will equip you with the knowledge and practices you need to appreciate this incredible stage of life.

So, take a deep breath, prepare to connect with your body and baby, and join me on this journey of self-care, rejuvenation, and empowerment via pregnancy yoga practice.

CHAPTER 1.

BENEFITS OF YOGA DURING PREGNANCY.

Pregnancy is a life-changing experience for women, with both physical and emotional changes. Maintaining both physical and emotional well-being is critical at this critical period, and yoga provides a holistic way to doing so. Yoga during pregnancy is becoming increasingly popular, and for good reason. It offers numerous advantages that lead to a healthier, more comfortable pregnancy and a more seamless transition into motherhood.

Yoga poses or asanas gently stretch and strengthen the body, aiding in the relief of common pregnant discomforts such as back pain and muscular tightness. These exercises are intended to enhance flexibility and balance, making it easier to adjust to the physical changes that come with pregnancy.

•**Improved Posture:** MAintaining proper posture as the belly expands can be difficult. Yoga promotes good alignment, which can help avoid spine strain and alleviate discomfort caused by poor posture.

•**Regulated Breathing:** Yoga emphasizes regulated breathing techniques. Learning to breathe deeply and mindfully during labor and delivery can be life-changing. These strategies help to alleviate discomfort and anxiety while also increasing oxygen supply to the developing baby.

•**Stress Reduction:** Pregnancy, especially for first-time mothers, can be stressful. Yoga encourages relaxation through meditation and awareness, which reduces tension and anxiety. This emotional equilibrium is advantageous not just to the mother but also to the developing fetus.

•Improved Circulation: The postures and movements of yoga promote blood circulation throughout the body. This can help to reduce swelling in the extremities, which is typical during pregnancy, as well as support general cardiovascular health.

•Weight Gain Can Be Controlled: While weight gain is normal during pregnancy, yoga can help limit excessive weight gain by supporting healthy eating habits and physical activity.

Yoga can help with typical aches and pains like lower back pain, sciatica, and leg cramps. Stretching and strengthening activities target and relieve trouble areas.

•Preparation for Labour: Certain yoga positions, including squatting and pelvic floor movements, can help prepare the body for labor and delivery by increasing pelvic flexibility and strength.

Yoga promotes focus and insight with your baby. During prenatal yoga classes, mothers frequently report feeling more connected to their developing baby, building a deeper emotional attachment.

•**Social Support:** Attending prenatal yoga courses allows expectant women to interact with other expectant mothers. Sharing one's thoughts and experiences can be soothing and help to build a supportive community.

Postnatal yoga builds on the basis of prenatal yoga, allowing for a faster recovery after childbirth. Strengthening the core and pelvic muscles might help the body recover from pregnancy.

•Emotional Resilience: Hormonal variations during pregnancy might impact mood. Yoga teaches women emotional strength and coping techniques that will help them manage these transitions more graciously.

•Improved Sleep: Many pregnant women have sleep difficulties. Yoga's relaxing practices can enhance sleep quality, ensuring that expectant moms get enough rest.

•Reduced Risk Of Gestational Diabetes: According to some research, practicing yoga during pregnancy may lower the risk of developing gestational diabetes, a disorder that affects blood sugar levels during pregnancy.

Yoga is more than simply physical exercise; it is a holistic approach that considers the mind, body, and spirit. This all-encompassing approach can result in a more balanced and enjoyable pregnancy experience.

Finally, there are numerous advantages to practicing yoga when pregnant. It promotes both the physical and emotional well-being of mother and child, resulting in a harmonious atmosphere for the baby's growth and development. However, before beginning any new fitness plan during pregnancy, it is critical to speak with a healthcare expert to confirm safety and suitability for unique circumstances.

Yoga, when practiced carefully and under competent supervision, can be a wonderful companion on the amazing journey of pregnancy.

CHAPTER 2.

PREPARING FOR YOUR YOGA PRACTICE.

Yoga, an ancient practice that unites the mind, body, and spirit, has grown in popularity in recent years due to its numerous health advantages. Whether you're a seasoned yogi or a newbie taking your first steps onto the mat, effective preparation is critical for a rewarding and safe yoga practice.

Yoga practice preparation is a combination of physical, mental, and environmental aspects that can considerably improve your experience. In this post, we'll look at the most important parts of preparation for a successful yoga practice.

1. Select the Appropriate Time and Location: The first step in planning for your yoga practice is to find a suitable time and location. Yoga is most effective when practiced at a time when your natural energy levels are in sync. Many people find that practicing in the morning gives them a boost of energy to start their day, whereas others prefer a relaxing evening practice to unwind after a long day. Regardless of the time of day, make sure your chosen location is calm, clutter-free, and well-ventilated. A dedicated yoga location can aid in the creation of ritual and regularity in your practice.

2. Wear Comfortable Clothes:

Your yoga practice can be considerably influenced by the clothes you wear. Choose clothing that is comfortable, breathable, and stretchy, allowing for a full range of motion. Tight or constrictive clothing can impede mobility and distract you from the awareness that yoga promotes. Consider the temperature of your practice area as well. Layers can assist you adjust to fluctuations in body temperature while practicing.

3. Gather Your Yoga Equipment:

While yoga may be practiced with minimal equipment, having the appropriate props can substantially improve your practice. A yoga mat is required for a solid and padded surface. Blocks, belts, and bolsters can help with appropriate alignment and comfort in a variety of poses. Having these things accessible can help you avoid distractions while practicing.

4. Hydrate and Feed Your Body:

A successful yoga practice requires proper hydration and nourishment. Drink water throughout the day to stay hydrated, but avoid big amounts shortly before practise to avoid discomfort. When it comes to food, it's preferable to practice yoga on an empty stomach, or with a little snack if needed. A large meal can make you feel lethargic and uneasy during your workout.

5. Make a Decision:

Take a moment to create an intention before beginning your physical practice. This can be a term, phrase, or thought that directs and aligns your practice with your aims and requirements. It could be anything as simple as "peace" or "strength." Setting an intention on the mat helps you stay focused and present.

6. Preparation:

Warming up is essential for avoiding injury and preparing your body for more challenging yoga poses. Begin with easy exercises such as neck rolls, shoulder rolls, and spinal twists. Gradually proceed to greater movements that include a variety of muscle groups. Warming up improves flexibility through increasing blood flow, loosening muscles, and increasing blood flow.

7. Pay Attention to Your Breath : Throughout

your yoga practice, your breath will function as a guide. Keep a close eye on your breathing and aim for deep, controlled inhalations and exhalations. The breath not only helps you stay present and connected to your practice, but it also oxygenates your body. Yoga requires you to coordinate your movements with your breath.

8. Respecting Your Body : Honoring your body's limitations is one of the most important components of preparation for your yoga practice. Yoga is about working with your body to find balance, flexibility, and strength, not forcing it into poses. If a pose causes discomfort or agony, adjust it or avoid it entirely. Pay attention to your body and remember that progress takes time.

9. Relaxation and Savasana :

After the physical component of your practice, it's crucial to stretch gently and finish with Savasana (Corpse Pose). Savasana helps your body and mind to totally relax, allowing you to integrate the benefits of your practice and prepare for the return to regular life. It's a period of deep repose and silence.

10. Reflection and Gratitude:

Take a minute to reflect on your yoga practice when you finish it. What are your current physical, mental, and emotional states? Thank yourself for the time you've spent on yourself and your well-being. This period of introspection can help you take the positive energy from your practice throughout the rest of your day.

Preparing for your yoga practice entails more than simply rolling out your mat and striking a posture. It is a comprehensive strategy that considers physical, mental, and environmental variables. By focusing on these factors and developing a mindful habit, you may maximize the advantages of your yoga practice and feel increased well-being both on and off the mat.

YOGA PRACTICE, SAFETY CONSIDERATIONS.

Yoga, a practice that improves physical and internal well- being, is well- known for its multitudinous advantages. Still, like with any physical exertion, there are pitfalls if not approached with caution. It's critical to ensure your safety during your yoga practice in order to avoid injuries and reap the full benefits of this ancient fashion. This post will go over important safety aspects in yoga practice.

1. Speak with a Medical Professional : It's stylish to see a healthcare expert before beginning a yoga trip, especially if you have any beginning health enterprises or injuries. They can advise you on whether yoga is right for you and make recommendations grounded on your specific requirements.

2. Select the Stylish Yoga Class : Yoga comes in a variety of styles, ranging from moderate Hatha to severe Ashtanga. Choose a class that corresponds to your fitness position and goals.However, starting with a freshman's or moderate class can help you produce a firm foundation while avoidingover-exertion, If you are a freshman or have physical restrictions.

3. Interact with Your Yoga educator : It's critical to communicate well with your yoga educator. Inform them if you have any medical issues, injuries, or physical limits. This allows them to give changes or druthers
to acts that may be dangerous to you. An educated educator will value your candor and put your safety first.

4. Be apprehensive of your body's limitations: Yoga promotes tone- mindfulness and acceptance. While it's necessary to push yourself, it's also critical to honor your body's boundaries. Avoid pushing yourself too hard or aiming for perfection in your positions. Pain or pain is a cue to relax or change the disguise, not to force it.

5. The significance of Proper Alignment : The significance of proper alignment in yoga practice can not be exaggerated. Strain, overstretching, and damage can be affected from misalignment.

Pay close attention to your educator's alignment instructions, and use props similar as blocks or strips as demanded to attain perfect alignment in acts.

6. Acceptable Warm-Up : Warming up is necessary for preparing your body for yoga acts. Gentle stretches, common reels, and deep breathing help ameliorate blood inflow and inflexibility, lowering the liability of strains or sprains during more delicate acts.

7. Mindfully Breathe : Yoga places a high value on breath mindfulness. Breath control not only improves the effectiveness of acts but also aids in injury forestallment. rather of holding your breath, keep it steady and controlled throughout the practise. It can help you concentrate and reduce stress.

8. Make Good Use of Props : Yoga props similar to blocks, belts and bolsters can be relatively useful for perfecting your practice and icing your safety. Use them to modify acts or make them more accessible, especially if you are a neophyte or have physical restrictions.

9. Make Small Steps : Yoga is a trip, not an end point. Avoid trying delicate positions before understanding the fundamentals. Progress sluggishly and patiently. This system not only reduces the chance of detriment but also allows you to enjoy the process of tone- enhancement.

10. Pay Attention to Your Body : In yoga, your body is your stylish school teacher. Back out incontinently if a station feels unwelcome or painful. Discomfort isn't the same as the" stretching sensation" you may feel in some positions. Learn to tell the difference between the two, and in no way put your body in an uncomfortable situation.

11. Maintaining Hydration and Nutrition : Dehydration can vitiate performance and increase the liability of cramps or muscular injuries. Make sure you are duly doused before and after your practice. To avoid gastric pain during postures, practice yoga on an empty stomach or with a light snack if necessary.

12. Keep Your Mat in Mind : A yoga mat provides stability and bumper, but if not duly maintained, it can be a source of slips and falls. Check that your mat is clean, dry and free of wrinkles or crimps that could beget you to lose your balance.

13. Avoid Making Comparisons : Yoga is a particular trip, and each person's body is unique. Avoid comparing yourself to your classmates, especially on social media. rather of trying to imitate someone differently, practice, concentrate on your own advancement and tone-enhancement.

Eventually, safety enterprises are critical for a satisfying and injury-free yoga practice. Yoga should be a trip of tone- discovery, mending, and progress, and clinging to these safety principles will allow you to reap the benefits of yoga while minimizing the hazards.

Keep in mind that safety, tolerance, and tone-compassion are all essential factors of your yoga practice.

CHOOSING THE RIGHT MATERNITY WEAR

Choosing the correct maternity yoga attire is essential for expectant women who want to keep a healthy and active lifestyle during their pregnancy. To accommodate the changing demands of the body, maternity yoga gear should prioritize comfort, support, and flexibility. Here are some important factors to consider when choosing prenatal yoga clothing:

1.Comfort is Essential : A woman's body undergoes major changes during pregnancy. Look for pregnancy yoga gear composed of materials that are soft, breathable, and stretchy, such as cotton or moisture-wicking mixes. These fabrics are comfortable and allow you to move freely during your yoga practice.

2.Supportive Bras : A supportive, well-fitting maternal sports bra is necessary. It should provide excellent support for your changing bust size while still allowing you to move freely. Adjustable straps and wide bands can aid with weight distribution.

3.Elastic Waistbands: Choose maternity yoga pants or leggings with elastic waistbands that sit comfortably below your tummy. These patterns will not dig into your skin during postures and will fit your developing bulge.

4.Layering Options: Because yoga studios can vary in temperature, wear an outfit that allows you to layer. A pregnancy tank top paired with a light jacket or cardigan will help you adapt to changing weather conditions.

5.Stay Stylish: While comfort and functionality are important, don't let style suffer. Many brands sell beautiful pregnancy yoga attire that will make you feel confident and appealing while you practice.

6.Scale Up Gradually: While it may be tempting to buy larger sizes, consider maternity attire that fits your current size and gradually expands to accommodate your increasing belly. Look for products that can be adjusted, such as drawstrings or fold-over waistbands.

7.Breathability: Pregnancy can cause you to feel hotter than usual, so choose fabrics that wick moisture away from your skin and allow it to breathe. This will help you keep cool and comfortable while you practice.

8.Spend Wisely: Although high-quality maternity yoga wear is more expensive, it is an investment in your comfort and well-being throughout pregnancy. Pieces that are well-constructed are more likely to keep their shape and last throughout your pregnancy and beyond.

9.Read Reviews: Before purchasing pregnancy yoga wear, read reviews from other expectant women to gain insight into the fit, comfort, and durability of certain maternity yoga wear brands and designs.

Remember that every pregnancy is different, so be open to trying new styles and brands to see what works best for you.

The correct pregnancy yoga attire can significantly improve your comfort and enjoyment of prenatal yoga, allowing you to stay active and relaxed while you prepare for motherhood.

CHAPTER 3.

BASIC YOGA POSES FOR EXPECTING MOMS: GENTLE STRETCHES.

Pregnancy is a physically and mentally changing experience for any woman. As the body changes, it's critical to find methods to stay active, relaxed, and connected to your growing kid. Yoga provides a comprehensive method to reach this balance, notably through gentle stretches intended exclusively for pregnant women.

1. Cat-Cow stance: The Cat-Cow stance is excellent for gently mobilizing the spine and pelvis. Begin on all fours, inhale by arching your back like a cat, and exhale by dipping your belly down. This regular movement relieves lower back stress, which is prevalent during pregnancy.
2. Child's stance: This stance is great for stretching and relaxing. Kneel on the floor, then sit back on your heels, arms extended and

forehead resting on the ground. It relieves back, hip, and shoulder stiffness.

3. Butterfly Stretch: Sit on the floor and pull your feet together, allowing your knees to fall to the sides. Flap your knees up and down to simulate the wings of a butterfly. This stretch stretches the hips and groin.

4. Prenatal Sun Salutation: A modified Sun Salutation sequence is great for improving flexibility and circulation during pregnancy. It consists of mild motions such as forward folds, lunges, and backbends, all while focusing on your breath.

5. Supported Triangle Pose: Stand with your feet apart, bend at the hips, and support yourself with your hand on a chair or a wall. This pose stretches your torso's sides and encourages greater balance, which can be difficult as your center of gravity shifts.

6. Standing Forward Bend: Begin by standing with your feet hip-width apart and bending forward at the hips, leaving your arms to hang loosely. This pose might help to relieve lower back discomfort and promote relaxation.

7. Pelvic Tilts: Rock your pelvis back and forth on your hands and knees. This workout helps to strengthen your abdominal muscles, which might be beneficial during labor and delivery.

8. Wall Squats: Stand with your back to a wall and lower yourself into a squatting position. This pose strengthens your leg muscles and increases your endurance for childbirth.

9. Savasana (Corpse Pose): Finish your yoga session by lying on your back with your legs slightly apart and your arms relaxed by your sides in Savasana. To relax your thoughts and lessen tension, focus on deep, deliberate breathing.

Keep in mind that when practicing yoga while pregnant, safety comes first. Before beginning any new fitness plan, especially during pregnancy, always consult with your healthcare professional. In addition, pay attention to your body and alter poses as needed.

The goal is to nurture your body, prepare for childbirth, and cultivate a sense of inner serenity during this unique time. Expectant moms can embark on a journey of physical and emotional well-being that helps both themselves and their growing babies by using these simple stretches.

BREATHING TECHNIQUES.

Prenatal yoga emphasizes deep, diaphragmatic breathing, commonly known as "belly breathing." This approach promotes relaxation and stress reduction by increasing oxygen supply to both the mother and the developing baby.

•Expectant mothers are taught the "Ujjayi" breath, sometimes known as the "ocean breath." In this technique, you inhale and exhale through your nose while gently restricting the back of your throat. It helps to increase lung capacity, which can be useful during labor.

•Prenatal yoga promotes "breath awareness" to assist pregnant women in staying in sync with their changing bodies. This attentiveness becomes increasingly important as the baby grows and helps ease discomfort caused by altered breathing patterns.

•Combating Shallow Breathing: In the later stages of pregnancy, limited diaphragmatic space can result in shallow breathing. Prenatal yoga provides strategies to combat this, ensuring that both mother and baby get enough oxygen.

Finally, the emphasis on breathing techniques in prenatal yoga provides expectant moms with vital tools for a healthy and thoughtful pregnancy.

These strategies promote relaxation, reduce stress, and prepare women for the physical demands of labor, resulting in a more pleasant and positive delivery experience.

PRENATAL YOGA RELAXATION POSES.

Prenatal yoga, a gentle and deliberate practice geared to pregnant moms, consists of a number of poses designed to improve physical comfort and mental relaxation. Relaxation positions are unique among these, providing tremendous advantages to both the mother and her growing baby.

•**Savasana, often known as the Corpse Pose: is** a popular relaxation pose in prenatal yoga. This supine position consists of resting on one's back, supported by cushions or bolsters beneath the head and knees. It promotes profound relaxation, allowing the mother to rest her body and mind.
•**Supta Baddha Konasana or Reclining Bound Angle Pose :** is another beneficial relaxation posture. In this position, the mother reclines with her feet together and her knees splayed outward. This mild stretch can help to relieve lower back pain and increase pelvic flexibility.

•**Balasana, or Child's Pose :** is a pregnant yoga pose that helps moms connect with their breath and reduce lower back strain. It promotes a forward fold with the knees apart, which supports the belly and provides a pleasant stretch.

These relaxation positions promote mental well-being as well as physical comfort. Prenatal yoga focuses on mindfulness and deep breathing, which assists moms in managing stress and anxiety throughout pregnancy.

Women are guided through these relaxation positions by prenatal yoga instructors, who ensure their safety and comfort. These poses, when practiced on a daily basis, contribute to a healthier pregnancy, less discomfort, and a more profound connection between the mother and her unborn child. The serenity and tranquility found in relaxation poses are vital gifts that resound far beyond the yoga mat on the maternal journey.

CHAPTER 4.

STRENGTHENING YOUR PELVIC FLOOR WITH PRENATAL YOGA.

Prenatal yoga is a holistic approach to preserving physical and emotional well-being throughout pregnancy, and one important component of this practice is pelvic floor strengthening. During pregnancy, the pelvic floor, a set of muscles that form a hammock-like structure at the base of the pelvis, plays an important function in supporting the expanding uterus and maintaining general pelvic health.

During pregnancy, hormonal changes and the baby's growing weight place additional strain on the pelvic floor. This can cause a variety of problems, such as urine incontinence, lower back pain, and even pelvic organ prolapse. Prenatal yoga is a safe and effective technique to deal with these issues.

Prenatal yoga positions emphasize moderate, controlled movements that assist develop the pelvic floor muscles. Breath control, relaxation, and flexibility are emphasized in these positions. Deep, conscious breathing is essential in prenatal yoga because it not only oxygenates the body but also encourages calm and connection to the pelvic region.

The Cat-Cow pose is one of the most often suggested poses for pelvic floor strengthening during pregnancy. This simple but effective practice improves pelvic flexibility and circulation while stimulating the pelvic floor muscles. Squats and hip-opening poses are also good because they promote pelvic mobility.

Prenatal yoga gives emotional support and stress alleviation in addition to physical benefits. Prenatal yoga sessions can provide expectant women with a sense of community and shared experience. These programmes frequently incorporate meditation and relaxation exercises, which can help women reduce anxiety and mentally prepare for labor and deliveries.

Prenatal yoga, in general, provides a comprehensive approach to pelvic floor wellness during pregnancy. Expectant moms can lower the risk of common difficulties and ensure a more comfortable pregnancy and birthing experience by strengthening these vital muscles. Furthermore, prenatal yoga's emotional and mental advantages lead to a sense of well-being that can assist both the mother and her growing baby.

UNDERSTANDING THE PELVIC FLOOR IN PRENATAL YOGA.

Expectant women can benefit from prenatal yoga, and understanding the pelvic floor is essential during this time. The pelvic floor is a collection of muscles, ligaments, and connective tissues that run along the bottom of the pelvis. The pelvic floor experiences considerable modifications during pregnancy to support the developing uterus and baby. Prenatal yoga can help women become more aware of and develop these muscles, resulting in a more comfortable pregnancy and childbirth.

First and first, awareness is essential. The importance of connecting with the pelvic floor is frequently emphasized in prenatal yoga classes. This awareness teaches expectant mothers how to engage and relax these muscles, which can be quite beneficial during labor.

Second, pregnant yoga regimens involve strengthening movements. These exercises are designed to increase pelvic floor strength without overexertion. Strong pelvic floor muscles can help support the baby's weight, alleviate discomfort, and improve posture throughout pregnancy.

Finally, flexibility exercises are essential. Yoga stretches and poses can help relieve pelvic tension and tightness. This greater flexibility may lower the likelihood of pregnancy problems such as pelvic pain or discomfort.

Prenatal yoga also teaches breathing methods. Breathing properly can help the pelvic floor function. Learning to breathe deeply and rhythmically throughout labor can help with relaxation and pain control.

Finally, prenatal yoga's pelvic floor exercises can help with postpartum rehabilitation. Stronger and more flexible pelvic floor muscles can help women restore bladder control and general core strength after childbirth.

In conclusion, prenatal yoga gives expectant mothers vital tools for understanding and caring for their pelvic floor. Yoga can help with a more comfortable pregnancy, an easier childbirth experience, and a faster postpartum recovery through increasing awareness, moderate strengthening, flexibility, and breathing methods. Prenatal yoga can boost physical and emotional well-being during pregnancy, ultimately benefiting both mother and baby.

PELVIC EXERCISES IN GESTATION YOGA .

Antenatal yoga is a peaceful and useful practice for pregnant women that involves multitudinous postures to enhance physical and emotional well- being throughout gestation.

Pelvic bottom exercises, in particular, are essential in antenatal

yoga programmes.

The pelvic bottom is a set of muscles that support the bladder, uterus, and rectum. Because of the expanding fetus, these muscles are put under adding strain throughout gestation. Pelvic bottom exercises, frequently known as Kegel exercises, help to strengthen and maintain the integrity of these muscles.

Antenatal yoga incorporates pelvic bottom exercises to address several main enterprises Pelvic bottom muscles atrophy during gestation due to hormonal changes and increased weight.

Through regulated condensation and releases, yoga assists women in engaging and strengthening these muscles :

•**Supporting the Uterus** : As the uterus develops, the pelvic bottom muscles keep it from drooping. Toned pelvic bottom muscles give important support to the expanding uterus, lowering the chance of problems.

•**Preventing Incontinence** : Numerous pregnant women develop urine incontinence. Pelvic bottom exercises enhance bladder control, minimizing leakage problems that are common during gestation and postpartum.

•**Enhancing Labour** : Strong pelvic bottom muscles can prop in the labor process. They prop in the descent of the baby through the delivery conduit and can make pushing more effective.

•**Postpartum Recovery :** Maintaining pelvic bottom health during gestation will help with postpartum recovery. These muscles are constantly injured during parturition, and preoperative strengthening can help to speed up mending.

Antenatal yoga courses are led by professional preceptors who lead actors through a series of pelvic bottom exercises. These generally number conscious breathing and controlled condensation of the pelvic muscles.

Yoga positions similar to Cat- Cow and Butterfly are also used to engage the pelvic bottom while developing inflexibility and relaxation. It's critical for awaiting mothers to check with their healthcare experts before commencing any fitness plan, including antenatal

yoga. They should also seek instruction from professional pregnant yoga preceptors to ensure that conditioning is completed rightly and securely.

In conclusion, the preface of pelvic bottom exercises within antenatal Yoga is a significant element of a holistic approach to pregnancy.

Expectant mothers can ameliorate their comfort throughout gestation, prepare for labor, and have a more comfortable postpartum recovery by strengthening these muscles.

MODIFIED YOGA POSES FOR PELVIC FLOOR HEALTH

Maintaining a strong pelvic bottom is essential for general well- being, and yoga can be a gentle yet effective approach to do it. There are some modified yoga positions that concentrate on strengthening and calming the pelvic bottom muscles.

•**Bridge Pose Variation :** Rest on your back with bent knees and flat feet , Lift your hips vocally off the bottom, cranking your glutes and pelvic floor muscles. Breathe deeply as you hold this station for numerous breaths.

•**Supine Bound Angle Pose :** Lie on your back, bend your knees, and bring the soles of your bases together. Allow your knees to drop to the sides, feeling a mild stretch in the inner shanks and pelvic area. Relax and breathe into this station.

•**Child's Pose with Wide Knees:** Begin in a kneeling position and spread your knees wider than hipsterism- range piecemeal. Sit back on your heels and extend your arms forward, allowing your forepart to rest on the ground. This position relieves pelvic strain.

•**Cat- Cow Pose :** Begin on your hands and knees in a tabletop position. Inhale as you arch your reverse(cow station) and exhale as you round your chine(cat disguise). This moderate movement improves pelvic inflexibility and rotation.

•**Modified Squat :** Stand with your bases wider than hipsterism- range piecemeal, toes turned slightly outside. sluggishly lower yourself into a thickset, maintaining your reverse straight and your hands at your heart center. This disguise develops the pelvic bottom and leg muscles.

•**Wide-Lawful Forward Fold :** Stand with your bases wide piecemeal. Depend on your hips and fold forward, allowing your upper body to hang. This position stretches the pelvic area gently while adding inflexibility.

•**Supported Bound Angle Pose :** Sit on a bumper or block, bend your knees, and bring the soles of your bases together. Gently press your knees against the bottom with your hands. This supported stretch is soothing.

Remember, it's important to listen to your body and never push yourself to the point of discomfort. Practicing these modified yoga poses regularly can contribute to better pelvic floor health over time. However, if you have any pelvic floor concerns or medical conditions, it's advisable to consult a healthcare professional before beginning a new exercise routine.

CHAPTER 5.

BOOSTING FERTILITY THROUGH YOGA.

Yoga is a holistic practice that can conceivably boost fertility by addressing physical, internal, and emotional aspects of well- being. While it's not a guaranteed answer, it can round medical fertility treatments and promote overall health. Then is how yoga can help fertility in 300 words

•**Stress Reduction** : Stress is a given cause that can negatively impact fertility. Yoga helps reduce stress through relaxation styles like deep breathing and contemplation. Lower stress situations can ameliorate hormonal balance and increase the chances of generality.

•Hormone Regulation : Certain yoga acts, similar as supported ground and cobra, stimulate the thyroid and pituitary glands, which play a crucial part in regulating hormones related to fertility.

•Improved Blood Circulation : Yoga promotes better blood inflow to the pelvic area. Poses like the butterfly disguise and the reclining set angle pose increase blood force to reproductive organs, conceivably enhancing their function.

•Enhanced Reproductive Organ Health : Yoga poses like the camel disguise and the chump disguise can help tone and strengthen the reproductive organs, conceivably perfecting their health and function.

•**Balancing The Endocrine System** : Yoga postures and breathing styles can help balance the endocrine system, which controls hormone products. This balance is important for fertility, as hormones impact ovulation and sperm production.

•**Body- Mind Connection** : Yoga supports a deeper connection between the mind and body. This heightened mindfulness can help people more understand their bodies and come more attuned to their fertility cycles.

•**Weight Management** : Operation Maintaining a healthy weight is important for fertility. Regular yoga practice can help in weight operation, which, in turn, can appreciatively impact fertility.

•**Emotional Well- Being :** Fertility problems can lead to emotional torture. Yoga's awareness and contemplation aspects can help people deal with the emotional challenges associated with gravidity, reducing the negative impact on fertility.

•**Increased Energy :** Yoga can boost energy situations and palliate fatigue, which can be helpful for couples trying to conceive.

•**Supportive Community :** Joining a yoga class can give a sense of community and internal support. participating with others who may be facing analogous fertility issues can be comforting.

While yoga can be a precious tool for enhancing fertility, it's important to approach it as a reciprocal practice alongside medical guidance. It may not guarantee generality, but it can contribute to a healthier body and mind, conceivably perfecting your chances of achieving your fertility pretensions. Always speak with a healthcare professional before starting any new exercise or heartiness routine, especially if you have underpinning health problems or are witnessing fertility treatments.

THE MIND- BODY CONNECTION.

Antenatal yoga is an awful way to nurture the mind- body link during gestation. It blends gentle physical postures, breath control, and contemplation to give several benefits

•**Physical Well- Being :** Antenatal yoga helps ameliorate inflexibility, balance, and strength, which can palliate typical gestation discomforts like reverse pain and lump.

•**Stress Reduction :** aware breathing and relaxation ways reduce stress and anxiety, supporting emotional well- being for both the mama and baby.

•**Bonding :** Yoga can produce a deeper connection between the mama and her growing baby, as it encourages awareness and a focus on the present moment. ,

•**Preparation for Labor :** Certain yoga acts and breathing exercises can be helpful in preparing the body for labor and delivery. They can ameliorate abidance and help with pain operations.

•Postpartum Recovery : The mind- body mindfulness formed during antenatal

Yoga can help in postpartum recovery and adaptation to fatherhood.

Flashback to speak with a healthcare provider before starting any new exercise program during gestation. It's essential to choose a pukka antenatal yoga educator who knows the specific requirements and safety considerations for pregnant women.

POSES TO ENHANCE FERTILITY.

Antenatal yoga is an awful practice for enhancing fertility, as it not only supports physical health but also reduces stress and increases overall well- being. While it's important to speak with a healthcare professional when trying to conceive, then are some yoga poses that may support fertility

•**Butterfly Pose (Baddha Konasana) :** This disguise stretches the groin and inner legs, promoting better blood inflow to the pelvic area.

•**Legs Up the Wall Pose (Viparita Karani):** This restorative disguise helps ameliorate rotation in the pelvic area and reduces stress.

•**Bridge Disguise Pose (Setu Bandhasana) :** It improves the pelvic muscles and can help balance hormones.

•Supine Twist (Supta Matsyendrasana) : Twists massage and detoxify internal systems, including the reproductive system.

•Pelvic Tilts : This simple practise can strengthen the pelvic muscles and ameliorate rotation.

•Meditations and Deep Breathing : Incorporating awareness and deep breathing styles into your practice can reduce stress and increase relaxation, which is important for fertility. Flash back that yoga alone may not guarantee fertility, but when combined with a healthy life, a balanced diet, and medical guidance, it can be a useful tool in your trip toward generality.

Always consult with a healthcare provider before starting any new exercise authority, especially if you are hoping to come pregnant.

CHAPTER 6.

YOGA SEQUENCES FOR EACH TRIMESTER.

Prenatal yoga can provide several benefits to both the mother and the growing fetus throughout the first trimester of pregnancy. This type of yoga focuses on gentle, pregnancy-safe poses and breathing methods that are customized to the specific needs of pregnant moms.

Prenatal yoga can help ease symptoms such as morning sickness and exhaustion throughout the first trimester. It encourages relaxation and reduces tension, both of which are necessary for a healthy pregnancy. Gentle stretching and strengthening activities promote flexibility, balance, and posture, which is especially important when the body changes rapidly.

Prenatal yoga breathing techniques increase lung capacity and oxygenate the body, benefiting both her and baby. They also help moms prepare for the controlled breathing that is essential during labor. Yoga also promotes emotional well-being by encouraging a connection between the mother and her growing baby.

Choosing a certified prenatal yoga instructor is critical during the first trimester since safety is vital. They may instruct expectant mothers on how to adapt postures to accommodate their changing bodies while also providing a safe and supportive environment.

In conclusion, prenatal yoga throughout the first trimester can be a beneficial technique for boosting physical and emotional well-being, alleviating pregnant pain, and preparing for a healthy labor and delivery experience. Before beginning any new workout plan during pregnancy, always consult with a healthcare physician to confirm it is appropriate for your specific circumstances.

SECOND TRIMESTER.

Prenatal yoga becomes a helpful practice for expectant moms throughout the second trimester of pregnancy. This phase, which normally lasts from weeks 14 to 27, brings with it changes and problems that prenatal yoga can effectively address.

Physically, the second trimester typically sees a decrease in morning sickness and a rise in energy levels. Prenatal yoga assists expectant mothers in maintaining and improving their flexibility, balance, and strength. Gentle poses and stretches alleviate typical aches and pains such as back pain and swollen ankles. It also helps to prepare the body for labor and delivery by emphasizing pelvic floor muscles and good breathing methods.

The second trimester can be an emotional time of greater confidence and connection with the growing baby. Through meditation and deep breathing exercises, prenatal yoga promotes calm and mindfulness. It offers a safe place for pregnant women to express their experiences and worries.

Prenatal yoga practice throughout the second trimester enhances physical comfort, mental well-being, and a stronger connection to the pregnancy experience. However, before beginning any fitness plan during pregnancy, it is critical to contact a healthcare expert to confirm that it is safe and appropriate for particular circumstances.

THIRD TRIMESTER.

Prenatal yoga is designed to help a pregnant woman's changing body and prepare her for childbirth throughout the third trimester. This phase, which normally lasts from weeks 28 to 40, necessitates extra care and changes.

The emphasis in the third trimester switches to mild stretching, deep breathing, and relaxation exercises. Poses are designed to alleviate discomfort, increase flexibility, and promote ideal fetal posture. Cat-Cow stretches, for example, relieve back stiffness, while pelvic floor exercises prepare for labor.

Breathing exercises become critical for dealing with labor contractions. Techniques such as Ujjayi breath and deep belly breathing promote relaxation and are useful for pain management.

However, safety comes first. Deep backbends, severe twists, and positions that compress the abdomen should be avoided by pregnant women. It is critical to stay hydrated and listen to one's body in order to avoid overexertion.

Prenatal yoga provides not only physical but also mental preparedness. It promotes a sense of community among expecting women while also reducing stress. Always with a healthcare physician before commencing any pregnant workout plan to ensure that it is compatible with individual health and pregnancy conditions.

CHAPTER 7.

YOGA FOR COUPLES.

Yoga for couples is a practice that promotes physical, emotional, and spiritual connection between lovers. The benefits of yoga are combined with the intimacy of a shared experience.

Yoga for couples consists of a series of partner positions and synchronized breathing techniques. These postures frequently necessitate trust and communication, which strengthens the link between partners. Couples can improve their physical flexibility and balance while also improving their emotional connection by using synchronized exercises and mindful breathing.

Yoga promotes awareness and reduces stress by encouraging couples to be present in the moment. It creates an environment for open conversation and mutual support.

Furthermore, the physical touch included in partner yoga might cause the release of oxytocin, the "love hormone," which promotes emotions of attachment and intimacy.

Overall, couples' yoga is a great method to strengthen your relationship, improve your physical health, and establish a harmonious connection between you and your partner. It's an opportunity to share a meaningful and rewarding experience that helps both the body and the heart.

CONNECTING WITH YOUR PARTNER.

Yoga is a lovely method for pregnant parents to connect on a deeper level during their pregnancy. It promotes emotional and spiritual bonding in addition to physical training.

Yoga allows partners to have a unique experience while also deepening their bond. Couples can create an intimate ambiance by synchronized breathing and soft positions, boosting their knowledge of each other's needs and feelings.

Furthermore, prenatal yoga allows for open dialogue. It helps partners to talk about their hopes, worries, and joys of parenthood, fostering understanding and support. Yoga's physical aspects, such as partner postures and massages, promote trust and teamwork, which are essential skills for parents.

The joint dedication to prenatal yoga provides a good example for future co-parenting. It reminds couples that they are a team on an incredible adventure together. This shared experience can serve as a basis for addressing the challenges and joys of motherhood together, deepening and expanding the link between couples as they approach this new era of life.

COUPLE BONDING POSES.

Prenatal yoga provides fantastic opportunities for expectant couples to bond. Here are some stances to help you connect:

•**Partner Breathing:** Sit cross-legged, holding hands, facing each other. Close your eyes, synchronize your breathing, and concentrate on the bond between you and your kid.

•**Assist with Child's Pose:** The mother assumes Child's Pose as the partner softly rubs her back and shoulders, promoting physical closeness and relaxation.

•**Standing Together:** Face each other and place your hands on your belly. Feel the baby's movements with him or her, creating a sense of shared expectancy.

•**Squat back-to-back:** while supporting each other's weight. This pose can help to strengthen the legs while also encouraging communication and teamwork.

•**Seated Twist:** Sit cross-legged, hold hands in opposite directions, and gradually twist. This increases spinal flexibility and the sensation of being in tune.

Sit comfortably with your partner and meditate together. Concentrate on your relationship and the new life you're bringing into the world.

During pregnancy, these positions encourage emotional bonding, physical support, and mindfulness, enhancing the connection between partners as they prepare for parenting. Remember to seek the advice and safety of a prenatal yoga instructor.

CHAPTER 8

YOGA FOR POSTPARTUM RECOVERY.

Yoga is a gentle and effective postpartum healing technique. Begin with simple poses like cat-cow and pelvic tilts to strengthen and relax the core. Gradually graduate to more advanced postures, keeping your body's restrictions in mind. Deep breathing exercises can help new mothers relax and minimize tension.

Yoga can help with postpartum healing by improving posture, relieving back discomfort, and increasing flexibility. It also encourages mother-baby bonding through gentle, baby-friendly positions. Always get the advice of a healthcare physician before beginning any workout plan following labor, and consider postpartum yoga courses for expert instruction.

SUPPORTING YOUR BODY AFTER BIRTH

Prenatal yoga is a fantastic approach to help your body recover after childbirth. It has several advantages for postpartum healing.

For starters, it strengthens the core muscles, which can weaken during pregnancy and labor. These strengthened muscles contribute to the restoration of abdominal strength and stability.

Second, prenatal yoga helps relaxation and stress reduction. Deep breathing methods taught in prenatal yoga can be used to cope with the stresses of new parenthood.

It can also help with common postpartum discomforts such back pain and muscular tension. Gentle stretches and poses help to reduce stress and increase flexibility.

Furthermore, it promotes emotional well-being. Yoga can help with postpartum anxiety and depression.

Finally, prenatal yoga promotes the mother-baby bond. Through soothing movements and gentle touch, it promotes bonding with your newborn.

In conclusion, doing prenatal yoga not only promotes physical recovery but also emotional and psychological well-being, making it an excellent choice for women on their postpartum journey.

Without a doubt, the following are the five most crucial ;

POSTPARTUM YOGA POSES

Balasana (Child's Pose): This pose gives relaxation and moderate stretching, making it great for reducing stress and soothing the mind.

Bridge Pose (Setu Bandha Sarvangasana): This pose strengthens the pelvic floor and back while boosting circulation, which is essential for postpartum recovery.

Pelvic Tilts: Important for regaining core strength and stability after childbirth.
Savasana: A relaxing pose that improves mental and physical recovery by reducing stress.

Cat-Cow Stretch: Excellent for improving spinal flexibility and alleviating tension in the back and neck, as well as promoting postpartum posture.

These postures target important components of postpartum recovery such as relaxation, core strength, pelvic health, and overall well-being. However, it is critical to practice them under adequate supervision and to pay attention to your body's needs.

SUMMARY AND CONCLUSIONS.

Finally, the practice of simple Yoga For Pregnancy, with a focus on pelvic floor postures, provides a holistic approach to boosting fertility and supporting expecting moms on their path to motherhood. These gentle yet effective yoga positions offer a plethora of benefits that can greatly improve a woman's chances of conception while also supporting general well-being throughout pregnancy.

The pelvic floor poses in this yoga routine, first and foremost, aim to strengthen the pelvic muscles. A strong pelvic floor is necessary for fertility because it supports reproductive organs, aids in uterine alignment, and promotes good blood circulation to the pelvic region. Women can establish a more friendly environment for conception by improving strength and flexibility in this area.

Furthermore, simple yoga for pregnancy emphasizes stress reduction and relaxation practices. Stress is a well-known element that can have a negative impact on fertility, and yoga is an excellent way to reduce stress levels. Expectant mothers can effectively manage stress by introducing deep breathing exercises, meditation, and mild stretches into their routine, promoting hormonal balance and boosting the likelihood of conception.

The mind-body connection developed by yoga is also important in increasing fertility. Women can become more attentive to their reproductive windows by growing knowledge of their bodies and cycles, making it simpler to time conception attempts efficiently.

This increased awareness empowers women to take charge of their reproductive health.
Simple yoga for pregnancy promotes general physical fitness and vitality.

Maintaining a healthy body weight and lifestyle is critical for fertility, and these yoga positions assist women in doing so. They promote healthy circulation, improve digestion, and relieve common pregnancy discomforts such as back pain and edema.

Furthermore, this practice promotes a supportive community of pregnant women who can share their stories, offer advice, and provide emotional support throughout the conception and pregnancy journey. This sensation of belonging may be both comforting and empowering.

Finally, simple yoga for pregnancy, with a focus on pelvic floor postures, provides a natural, accessible, and all-encompassing approach to improving fertility and supporting overall well-being for expecting mothers.

This yoga practice provides women with vital tools to optimize their chances of conceiving while nourishing their bodies and minds throughout pregnancy by strengthening the pelvic floor, lowering stress, boosting the mind-body connection, and encouraging physical health.

Embracing this holistic approach to parenthood can empower women and lay the groundwork for a joyful journey ahead.